Terminal Child

A Sister's Experiences

I0481623

Annabelle
Kimbrough

Annabelle Kimbrough
TERMINAL CHILD

Acknowledgements

To Rhonda Branch Yearby-A Very Special thank you for being my writing coach, & publisher and treating and loving me like your own grand-daughter. I love you.

Candi Rodgers- Special thank you for being an awesome teacher who cared about me, and loved me like a daughter. I love you.

Doctors who cared for my brother, Jesse- Special thank you for taking such good care of him, and working with us through bad times and the good times. I love you.

Jesse Kimbrough- Special thank you for being my brother, and giving me the opportunity of a lifetime to be able to have experienced having a terminally sick sibling.

Annabelle Kimbrough
TERMINAL CHILD

Table of Contents

Chapter 1

Birth

Before I was even thought of, my mom was pregnant with my older brother, Jesse. She almost miscarried 4 times before he finally came a month premature. I was born 15 months later. My first trip with my family, was a doctor visit for Jesse in Dallas, Texas, 2 weeks later. My family and I made several different trips that I don't even remember because I was too young. The first trip that I remember, was to New Orleans when I was 9 months old and into everything. I played with Mrs. Violet's trinkets because I thought they were cool. I would put toys and other things all over her house, but she didn't care, because she had grandkids of her own.

They lived beside her and I got to play with them, or I thought I was playing with them. They were older than me, so they were playing with me. When we walked back over to Mrs. Violet's house, she had good southern food cooked for us, for supper. The next few days, I stayed at the house with her when my parents would take Jesse to his doctor visits. That was his first trip there, so they were trying to figure out what was wrong with him.

I just thought he was my brother and that we went on a trip for fun. I was a little kid, so going on a trip was fun. But eventually, as I was getting older, and so was he, he got worse. More doctor visits came into our lives and I was drug here, there, and yonder with my family because they were trying to keep Jesse alive. I didn't understand why he was acting weird all the time, but I knew something must have been wrong the way everyone was so busy with Jesse.

He was always getting attention but not me. I felt lonely and I was sad, and didn't understand. As I got older, my parents would say stuff about him and what would be happening. I was old enough to understand that he was very sick. My little brother Samuel, was born 3 and ½ years later. By that time, the doctors were figuring out some of Jesse's issues, and so of course Samuel was the new born baby, so he got a lot of attention too. Too me, I felt like I was pushed aside again. It's not that I wasn't loved, it was just he was a new baby and could not survive on his own. It made me feel unwanted because Samuel and Jesse both received all my parent's attention and I was just set aside like I wasn't as important as they were.

Chapter 2

Stable

More Family Time

Even though Jesse was stable, his health problems were worse than what was expected. He was always having issue. Some of Jesse's issues were solved with medication. We were able to relax after 4 years of his life, because he got his feeding tube. We were able to do more family things, but they had to be things he could do too. When I was 4 years old, I played tee-ball. I played until I was 6 years old. My little brother Samuel played wee-ball when he was 3.

Jesse was always there with us to watch us play. He would laugh and cheer us on in his own language, because he couldn't talk. Then when I was about 7, I played softball. It always took several minutes to unload him and all of us and our equipment, and the same to load back up. It was a lot of work, but it was fun. Jesse was still dong good health wise.

When he was 8 years old, he had tendon release surgery on his groin, knees, and his ankles. He was in the hospital for a week. He had casts on both legs for several months. I could help my parents take care of him. He couldn't do anything for himself, not even sit up. It made me feel good knowing I got to help "my baby". Yes, I called him "my baby", because I took care of him, and he was just like a baby. He had Duchenne Muscular Dystrophy and several other health disorders. He wasn't even supposed to be alive, but he was.

Chapter 3

How It Made Me Feel

I loved my brother and everything, but his health problems or his mental disorder was so severe that there was no reason for h m to be living. My dad always would tell us that the doctors said Jesse defied science and medicine, and that the only reason for h m to be alive was because of God. I felt cool having a brother like Jesse, but I also felt different. Everywhere we went, people would always stare, which made me uncomfortable. I don't know why people would look at us like we didn't belong. I guess they feared Jesse. But why fear him?

He was harmless, and he loved everybody. My dad always told us that Jesse was a player because he had so many girlfriends. When Jesse would see any of his girlfriends, he would just start smiling and going crazy happy. Jesse was easy to like and love. He was always smiling, even when he was hurting. In my opinion, he was the happiest human being you would ever meet in the whole world. He couldn't physically come out and say that he loved us, but we knew he did because of how he was around us or anyone he met. He looked at everyone with love in his eyes and he would show his love or say he loved us in his own special ways.

Even though some people feared him, because they didn't know him, or some people would make fun of him, he was still my older brother and I wasn't going to let them stop me from being proud to have a brother like Jesse. He was a miracle baby and no other babies will ever be like him.

Chapter 4

Life Throughout School

Kids at school would laugh and make fun of Jesse because he was in a wheelchair, and would also make fun of me because I was related to him. I tried to ignore them but sometimes it didn't work. I would go home feeling like crap. I never stopped loving him though, because he couldn't help the way he was. Life throughout school, for us, wasn't always being bullied. He started having seizures often during school and would be checked out of school and go to the hospital. My little brother Samuel and I would then have to go to the after-school activity club thing, so we had somewhere to go.

My parents were friends with the owners, so we got to go for free because of the situations with Jesse being at the hospital. The other kids there, kind of stayed away from us, as if we were diseased or something; so, we just watched the other kids have fun. We wanted to have fun with the other kids, but it was hard if no one wanted to be your friend. Samuel eventually got to go play with the other kids, because he always made friends easy. To this day, he still does, and is in with the popular kids at school. I was worried about Jesse, so I was kind of too sad to play games with the other kids.

The seizures happened a lot throughout school, so we went to the after-school club thing a lot. When we would all go to New Orleans for his regular doctor appointments, we usually were given tickets to the Zoo and the Aquarium, so our trips were not always doctors, doctors, and, doctors; we had fun as well, which was a good thing. The hospital we went to had amazing food, and I don't usually like hospital food because it is nasty. The trips to New Orleans were usually a week long, so we were all tired by the time it was time to head home. It didn't bother me though, because I knew I could sleep on the way back home.

Chapter 5

Life in High School

When I reached 9th grade, and Samuel was in 8th grade, we were put in online school called "K12 Online Public School". Jesse was in 10th grade in regular school, but he reached the point where he was too sick to stay in school, so my parents pulled him out. Jesse had a teacher that would come to our house, so he could still learn, he just wouldn't be around kids at school that came up there even when they were sick. On his last doctor visit, which we didn't realize it was his last until we left, they told us his spine was curving forward and his diaphragm was being pushed up, which was putting pressure on his lungs.

They gave us an appointment card for his 18th birthday after that visit, and I told my dad, "hey, that's Jesse's 18th birthday". My dad told the doctor and the nurses that it was his birthday and that they should throw him a birthday party. They then looked at us with a "dead deer in the headlights" look, and so we walked out. On the way home, we realized that the appointment card was just to give us hope for our long, 6-hour drive home; which to us felt like a lifetime worth of driving home. That was when it hit me that my brother was about to die. I started posting on Facebook about it, so everyone knew what was happening.

My dad started getting lots of phone calls about it and could barely focus on his driving because of all the phone calls. 3 and ½ months later, on October 31st, Jesse's home health nurse was putting him in the bathtub, and he screamed out. We didn't know what happened, and went running down the hallway to see what was wrong. My dad scooped up Jesse and carried him to his bed and got him calmed down and put him to bed for a nap. Later that evening, we had our friends over for supper, and my dad told my mom that they needed to check on Jesse and so my dad went and checked on him. He started yelling, "Ginny! Ginny!

Get in here now!". Everyone went running in there, and Jesse's face was as white as a ghost, and his lips were a bluish-purple color.

My dad called 911, and my mom called some of her friends and her mom. They all came to join us around Jesse while waiting on 911 to get there. When they finally arrived, they checked on Jesse to see if he was okay, and one of the paramedics got in my moms' face about transporting Jesse to the hospital, but my mom fought back.

The lady paramedic kept pushing and so my mom's friend, Cheri Nash, stepped in between my mom and the lady paramedic without realizing it, and then the lady shut up because she saw that she better not messes with my mom because she was like a mother bear protecting her cub. They got Jesse settled down again for the night, so everyone then left.

The next morning, Jesse's eyes were fixed and dilatated. It was like he was in coma, only his eyes were open and moving back and forth. My dad got a flashlight to check his eyes and they were huge, so my dad called Jesse's doctor and they told him, "who knows how much longer Jesse has left; maybe seconds, hours, days, months; so, we needed to spend some time with him before he died". It was like 5 minutes after he got off the phone with the doctor that he went to the fire station because he accidentally gave them the nurses stethoscope, the night before. About 10 minutes later, after my dad left, Samuel was in his bedroom, my mom and I were in Jesse's room, and the nurse and her supervisor were outside talking. Jesse came out of the coma type thing and he turned his head at my mom and moaned at her as if he was saying he loved her and that everything was okay and goodbye.

My mom yelled for Samuel to come in there to us, and then Jesse took his last breath. I ran outside and got his nurse and her supervisor, and they both came inside and checked for a pulse, but could not find one. My mom called my dad and told him, and he came home. They called the deputies and the coroner. The deputies had to question my parents and the nurses because he died at home, and then the coroner pronounced him dead, so the funeral home came and got him. My parents then rushed everyone out of our house and we went to Celebrate Recovery, at our church.

Chapter 6

The Funeral and the Rest of My School Year

On November 5, 2013, we had Jesse's funeral. We had so many people there, that I felt kind of overwhelmed. Our family had to sit in a special section, but I wanted some of our friends to sit with me, so they did. It made me feel better to have our friends there with me. To be honest, I didn't know how or what to feel about my brothers passing. It just didn't feel real and still doesn't at times. I am still kind of numb to his passing. School was hard for Samuel and me because we gave up our school work when he died.

I had to do 10th grade twice. I became really depressed and started to self-harm. I started having suicidal thoughts and my anger has been bad since he passed, more so than it has ever been in my whole life. One of my teachers this past year, in 2017, right before I graduated, I told her everything about what happened with Jesse and how I became really depressed and everything. She cared about me and how I felt. She reached out to me with open arms, and it felt like she loved me. She started talking to me and was trying to help me through that bad situation. I was telling her how close I was to giving up on my life because of how bad I missed my brother and was so emotionally exhausted from a l the bullying I went through with my brother and me, and then losing him, was the worst pain I had ever felt. My teacher was the first person I opened to. I am not going to say her name because I don't want to cause any issues. Thank you for helping me, and I love you. You are like a mom to me, and you know who you are.

Prayers for those who are Terminally Ill & their families

_____
_____
_____
_____
_____
_____
_____
_____
_____
_____
_____
_____
_____
_____
_____
_____
_____
_____
_____
_____
_____
_____
_____
_____

About the Author:

I have just graduated high school; May 8, 2017. I'm not sure what I want to be anymore. I used to say I wanted to be a veterinarian, but I am searching different options available. I am passionate about drawing, singing, and riding horses. I love helping others and spreading the word of God, and his love for everyone. I have volunteered with Samaritan's Purse since 2016, and plan to do more. I want to help others feel better about themselves and want them to overcome their pasts. God loves all of you and will guide you where you need to go